Writing to Heal (Transformational) Journal

A Journey of Self-Discovery, Transformation & Inner Peace

Carlene Stanislaus

Dedication

I dedicate this transformational journal to every person who needs to heal from something-pain, abuse, or trauma. Whatever it is that you are seeking to obtain healing for, I sincerely hope that this journal will be a valuable tool to enable you to heal, transform, and evolve.

All healing is a process. What works for one individual may not necessarily work for another. It is up to you to decide and choose what resonates with you and where you are currently.

By choosing to heal today, you give yourself the opportunity to create the best version of yourself.

I also want to dedicate this journal to my dearest son, Sammy Orlando Bahous, who has been the equivalent of my right arm over the last 10 months of my life. Whilst I have been dealing with a near-death experience, which shook me to my core, I have fought every day to complete and publish this journal. Now that it is being published, I am forever grateful for this moment.

With heartfelt gratitude for my brother, Marlon Orlando Stanislaus, I give thanks for all his support and encouragement throughout my life.

Last but not least, Almighty God, it is by God's grace that I am alive today.

My intention going forward is to continue to create and write to help humanity to heal, transform, and evolve.

About the Author

Carlene Stanislaus, a devoted mother and author of *Writing to Heal*, her first book, is transforming lives all over the world. A certified professional in Life Coaching, mBIT, NLP, and Language and Behavior Profile, she seamlessly integrates spirituality with community service in the area of the healing arts. Carlene also holds certifications in Angelic Reiki to the Master Teacher level and as a Usui Reiki Master. These modalities of personal and professional development have been invaluable tools on her journey to date.

At this time in Carlene's life, she has answered the call of God and is pursuing ministry school studies. (Carlene also offers massage therapy to help uplift her community, which began as a hobby.)

Carlene enjoys singing, dancing, writing, and fitness, as well as actively embracing her faith, intimacy, and love for God.

Letter to the Reader

My Beloved Reader,

It is not by chance that you are holding this journal today. I do not believe in coincidences. Everything happens as it's supposed to.

(That does not mean that my beliefs are always correct, or that you need to believe in my beliefs.)

What matters is this: You chose this. You are choosing healing. You are choosing yourself.

Your decision to use this journal to heal, transform, and become the best version of yourself is one you will never regret. What you choose today affects your future and your future self will thank you.

As you begin this journey, ask yourself:

- What do you desire to feel healed from?
- What do you need to let go of?
- Who do you need to forgive?
- Do you need to forgive yourself?
- How would you like to feel once you've healed?
- Who would you like to become?
- What would you like your life to look like one year from today?

These questions are not about rushing to answers. They are about beginning a conversation with your soul. Take your time. Go gently. This journal is yours.

With love,

Carlene Stanislaus

How to Use This Journal

This journal is your sacred space.

There are no rules only gentle invitations.

You'll find:

• Exercises to explore your mind and body connection

• Prompts to guide self-reflection

• Pages to visualize and reimagine your story

• Blank spaces to rest, draw, or create your own rituals

You can go in order, skip ahead, or revisit pages as you grow.

You are the guide. Let your intuition lead.

Some days you might write four pages.

Other days, a single word may be enough.

There's no right way to do this only your way.

You may laugh.

You may cry.

You may discover something you didn't expect.

That's part of the process. Be patient with yourself.

Most importantly: **Be honest. Be kind. Be curious.**

Healing isn't about perfection.

It's about presence.

This journal is a companion, not a checklist.

Let it hold your mess and your magic alike.

Start where you are,

and let this journal meet you there.

Your Mind at a Glance

THE MIND

CONSCIOUS MIND

SUBCONSCIOUS MIND

BODY

- CHOOSE
- ACCEPT
- REJECT
- ORIGINATE

- MUST ACCEPT
- CANNOT REJECT
- CANNOT DIFFERENTIATE THE DIFFERENCE BETWEEN WHAT IS REAL AND WHAT IS IMAGINED

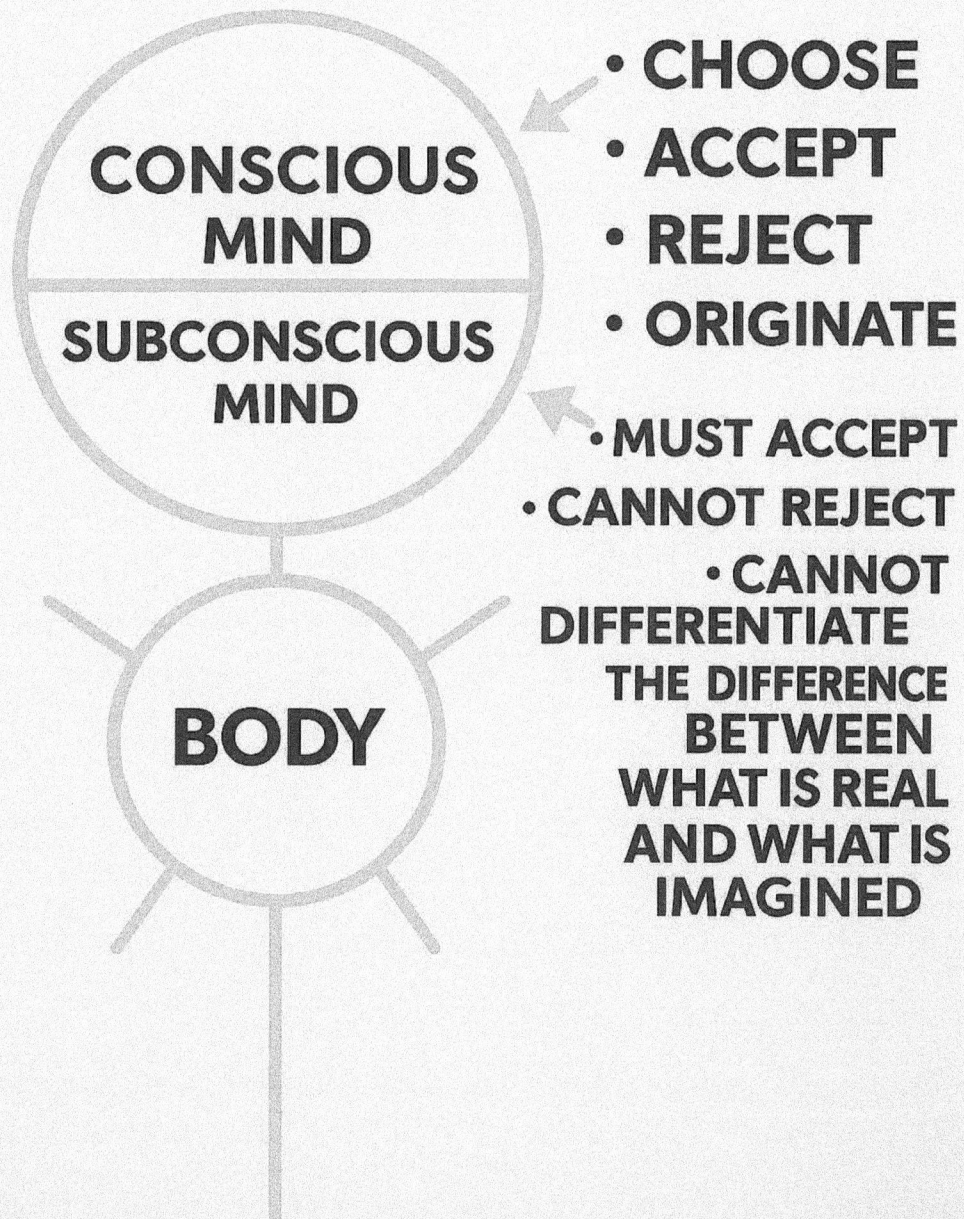

Credit: Dr. Thurman Fleet, San Antonio, Texas 1934

Conscious vs. Subconscious Mind

Two Parts, One Mind

The Conscious Mind

This is the part of your mind that you use when you're actively thinking, planning, judging, and analyzing. It's responsible for logic, short-term memory, decision-making, and awareness.

The voice says, "I should do this or this *makes sense.*"

The conscious mind is what we often identify with it's where our sense of self tends to reside moment to moment. The part of you which reads these words, forms opinions, and solves problems in real time.

But while the conscious mind is powerful, it only governs about 5% of your daily behavior. That means most of your reactions, habits, and emotional triggers are actually being guided by something deeper.

Understanding how your conscious mind operates is key to catching automatic thoughts and interrupting patterns. It allows you to pause, reflect, and choose rather than react.

Think of your conscious mind as the driver's seat. But remember: it still relies on the engine beneath the subconscious mind to move forward.

The more aware you become of your conscious thoughts, the more you can redirect your life with intention. Awareness is the first step in every transformation.

Even small shifts in conscious thought can ripple into lasting change.

It's where clarity begins and where healing choices are made.

When you observe your thoughts without judgment, you reclaim your power.

Your conscious mind is not just a thinker it's a doorway to change.

The Subconscious Mind

This is the deeper layer the part of your mind that runs the show behind the scenes. It holds your memories, beliefs, habits, patterns, and emotions.

It's not logical. It's emotional. And it doesn't respond to facts.

It responds to **repetition**, **emotion**, and **imagination**.

Think of the subconscious mind as a massive internal archive. Everything you've ever seen, heard, felt, or experienced is stored here even if you don't consciously remember it. It influences how you react to people, how you view the world, and how you treat yourself.

Many of your beliefs were planted here during childhood often without your awareness. These beliefs can quietly shape your sense of worth, your ability to trust, your fear of failure, or your fear of success.

The subconscious mind doesn't question what it holds. If it heard something repeatedly "I'm not good enough," for example it stores that as truth, even if it's harmful or outdated.

But here's the good news: what was once programmed can be reprogrammed. With intention, love, and practice, you can teach your subconscious mind new beliefs ones that support your healing and growth.

This journal is your first step in speaking to your subconscious mind with clarity, care, and compassion.

Your subconscious mind is always listening even when you're not speaking.

The stories you tell yourself today become the patterns you live tomorrow.

🦋 *The subconscious mind is where your healing begins because it's where your hurt was stored.*

3

Thoughts, Feelings & the Body

How the Mind Affects the Body

Every thought creates a feeling.

Every feeling creates a vibration in your body.

Over time, repeated emotions become your body's default state.

Stressful thoughts? You may feel tension, anxiety, or fatigue.

Empowering thoughts? You may feel light, calm, and energized.

The body listens. Always.

Your body is not separate from your mind it's a mirror. When your inner world is full of fear, grief, shame, or pressure, your body often absorbs it without question. You may notice it in clenched jaws, tight shoulders, shallow breathing, or digestive issues.

Likewise, when you begin to feel safe, loved, and grounded, your body responds. Your heart rate slows. Your muscles relax. You feel more open and present.

This is why awareness matters. When you change the messages you send to your mind, you also shift the chemical and energetic responses in your body.

You can begin healing not just by "thinking positively," but by **feeling intentionally** with compassion, truth, and consistency.

Use your body as a guide. It will tell you when something feels aligned… and when something needs love.

With practice, you can teach your body a new emotional language one rooted in safety, joy, and connection.

Your body remembers. But it can also relearn.

🦋 "What you think, you feel. What you feel, you become."

Programming the Subconscious Mind

Where Do Beliefs Come From?

Most of your subconscious mind beliefs were formed in childhood.

They come from:

• What you were told

• What you witnessed

• What you interpreted without fully understanding

As children, we absorb everything spoken and unspoken. We make meaning out of what we see, hear, and feel, often without context or logic. These early interpretations shape our core beliefs, sometimes in ways that limit us later in life.

These beliefs shape how you feel about:

• Yourself ("I'm not good enough" vs. "I am worthy")

• Others ("People will hurt me" vs. "I can trust again")

• The world ("It's dangerous" vs. "It's safe to grow")

The subconscious mind doesn't analyze it accepts. If something was repeated or emotionally intense, your mind stored it as truth.

But here's the powerful part: you don't have to keep living by beliefs that were never really yours. Beliefs are not permanent. They are learned and what was learned can be unlearned.

By becoming aware of your subconscious mind programming, you can begin to shift it with conscious intention.

Awareness is the first step.

Choice is the next.

Repetition is the key.

You are not stuck. You are teachable.

And your mind is ready to learn a new truth.

Identify Your Beliefs

What's living in Your Mind?

Instructions: Answer these questions honestly.

There are no right or wrong answers just awareness.

1. What beliefs did you grow up with about love?

_____

_____

_____

_____

_____

_____

_____

_____

_____

_____

_____

_____

_____

_____

_____

_____

_____

_____

_____

_____

2. What did you learn about emotions (e.g., crying, anger)?

_____

_____

_____

_____

_____

_____

_____

_____

_____

_____

_____

_____

_____

_____

_____

_____

_____

_____

_____

_____

_____

_____

3. Were your needs heard as a child?

_____

_____

_____

_____

_____

_____

_____

_____

_____

_____

_____

_____

_____

_____

_____

_____

_____

_____

_____

_____

_____

_____

4. What do you believe about your worth today?

_____

_____

_____

_____

_____

_____

_____

_____

_____

_____

_____

_____

_____

_____

_____

_____

_____

_____

_____

_____

_____

_____

_____

_____

5. When something goes wrong, what's the first thought you have?

_____

_____

_____

_____

_____

_____

_____

_____

_____

_____

_____

_____

_____

_____

_____

_____

_____

_____

_____

_____

_____

6. How do you talk to yourself when you make a mistake?

Healing & Transformation

You are the author of your healing.

In this section, you will be invited to reflect, release, and reconnect. The prompts ahead are not here to judge you. They are here to meet you exactly where you are.

Some may bring clarity. Others may stir emotion. That's okay. Healing isn't always easy but it is always worth it.

There's no need to rush or "get it right." You don't need to have the perfect words. You only need your truth.

Write honestly.

Write freely.

Write as if no one will ever read it because this is for you and you alone.

You can answer one prompt a day or revisit the same one over time.

Some pages may be blank. Some may be messy. All of it is healing.

Let your pen become your permission slip. Let your heart be loud on these pages, even if your voice is quiet elsewhere.

Don't be afraid of what comes up. Whatever surfaces, you're strong enough to face it and gentle enough to hold it.

This is your space.

Let it become sacred.

Let it become safe.

Let it become yours.

Healing is not a destination it's a relationship. With yourself. With your truth. With your future.

And it begins here.

"The wound is the place where the light enters you."

Rumi

Prompt:

What do you most want to heal from at this moment in your life?

Affirmation:

"Awareness is the beginning of transformation."

_____

_____

_____

_____

_____

_____

_____

_____

_____

_____

_____

_____

_____

_____

_____

_____

_____

_____

_____

_____

Prompt:

What have you been carrying for too long that you're ready to release?

Affirmation:

"I give myself permission to let go of what no longer serves me."

_____

_____

_____

_____

_____

_____

_____

_____

_____

_____

_____

_____

_____

_____

_____

_____

_____

_____

_____

_____

Prompt:

What emotions are you most afraid to feel? Why?

Affirmation:

"I am safe to feel. My emotions do not control me they guide me."

_____

_____

_____

_____

_____

_____

_____

_____

_____

_____

_____

_____

_____

_____

_____

_____

_____

_____

_____

_____

_____

Prompt:

Who or what has hurt you that still echoes in your mind?

Affirmation:

"I honor my pain. I am learning to move forward with compassion."

_____

_____

_____

_____

_____

_____

_____

_____

_____

_____

_____

_____

_____

_____

_____

_____

_____

_____

_____

_____

_____

Prompt:

What would forgiveness feel like in your body?

Affirmation:

"Forgiveness frees me, not them. I choose peace."

_____

_____

_____

_____

_____

_____

_____

_____

_____

_____

_____

_____

_____

_____

_____

_____

_____

_____

_____

Prompt:

In what ways have you abandoned or betrayed yourself to please others?

Affirmation:

"I return to myself with love and loyalty."

Prompt:

What limiting beliefs are running your life that no longer feel true?

Affirmation:

"I am not my past. I am allowed to choose again."

Prompt:

What would your life look like if you believed you were worthy?

Affirmation:

"I am worthy because I exist. I don't need to prove my value."

_____

_____

_____

_____

_____

_____

_____

_____

_____

_____

_____

_____

_____

_____

_____

_____

_____

_____

_____

_____

Prompt:

What do you most want your future self to remember about today?

Affirmation:

"Every moment is a seed. I choose to plant love and truth."

Prompt:

What would it feel like to be fully seen and accepted for who you are?

Affirmation:

"I am enough as I am. I welcome the love that sees the real me."

_____

_____

_____

_____

_____

_____

_____

_____

_____

_____

_____

_____

_____

_____

_____

_____

_____

_____

_____

_____

Prompt:

What does safety feel like in your body, mind, and soul?

Affirmation:

"It is safe for me to feel safe."

Prompt:

When do you feel most disconnected from yourself and why?

Affirmation:

"I come home to myself with patience and love."

_____

_____

_____

_____

_____

_____

_____

_____

_____

_____

_____

_____

_____

_____

_____

_____

_____

_____

_____

_____

_____

_____

Prompt:

What part of your past needs the most compassion?

Affirmation:

"I send love to the version of me who didn't know better."

_____

_____

_____

_____

_____

_____

_____

_____

_____

_____

_____

_____

_____

_____

_____

_____

_____

_____

_____

Prompt:

When was the last time you truly felt joy? What were you doing?

Affirmation:

"I deserve joy, and I invite more of it into my life."

_____

_____

_____

_____

_____

_____

_____

_____

_____

_____

_____

_____

_____

_____

_____

_____

_____

_____

_____

_____

_____

Prompt:

What message would you send to the younger version of yourself?

Affirmation:

"You did the best you could. I'm proud of you."

_____

_____

_____

_____

_____

_____

_____

_____

_____

_____

_____

_____

_____

_____

_____

_____

_____

_____

_____

_____

_____

_____

Prompt:

What is one truth you've been afraid to say out loud?

Affirmation:

"My truth is sacred. I honor it without shame."

_____

_____

_____

_____

_____

_____

_____

_____

_____

_____

_____

_____

_____

_____

_____

_____

_____

_____

_____

Prompt:

How do you define healing for yourself?

Affirmation:

"Healing is not a destination it is a relationship with myself."

_____

_____

_____

_____

_____

_____

_____

_____

_____

_____

_____

_____

_____

_____

_____

_____

_____

_____

_____

_____

_____

Prompt:

What are you still waiting for permission to do, say, or be?

Affirmation:

"I grant myself full permission to be all of me."

_____

_____

_____

_____

_____

_____

_____

_____

_____

_____

_____

_____

_____

_____

_____

_____

_____

_____

_____

_____

_____

Prompt:

What does freedom mean to you? Where do you feel trapped?

Affirmation:

"I am ready to set myself free."

Prompt:

What emotions have you inherited that don't belong to you?

Affirmation:

"I release what is not mine. I honor what is."

_____

_____

_____

_____

_____

_____

_____

_____

_____

_____

_____

_____

_____

_____

_____

_____

_____

_____

_____

Prompt:

What would it feel like to fully trust yourself?

Affirmation:

"I trust myself more with each breath."

Prompt:

What is one story you've told yourself that you're ready to rewrite?

Affirmation:

"I have the power to create a new narrative."

_____

_____

_____

_____

_____

_____

_____

_____

_____

_____

_____

_____

_____

_____

_____

_____

_____

_____

_____

_____

_____

Prompt:

Who inspires you and why?

Affirmation:

"I carry the strength of those who came before me."

_____

_____

_____

_____

_____

_____

_____

_____

_____

_____

_____

_____

_____

_____

_____

_____

_____

_____

_____

_____

_____

Prompt:

Where do you feel most at peace?

Affirmation:

"I return to the spaces that bring me calm."

_____

_____

_____

_____

_____

_____

_____

_____

_____

_____

_____

_____

_____

_____

_____

_____

_____

_____

_____

Prompt:

What relationship in your life needs clearer boundaries?

Affirmation:

"My boundaries protect my peace."

_____

_____

_____

_____

_____

_____

_____

_____

_____

_____

_____

_____

_____

_____

_____

_____

_____

_____

_____

Prompt:

What are you proud of even if no one noticed?

Affirmation:

"My worth is not measured by recognition."

_____

_____

_____

_____

_____

_____

_____

_____

_____

_____

_____

_____

_____

_____

_____

_____

_____

_____

_____

_____

Prompt:

What do you need to forgive yourself for?

Affirmation:

"I give myself the grace I so freely give others."

_____

_____

_____

_____

_____

_____

_____

_____

_____

_____

_____

_____

_____

_____

_____

_____

_____

_____

_____

_____

_____

Prompt:

What part of yourself have you hidden from the world?

Affirmation:

"My wholeness is welcome here."

_____

_____

_____

_____

_____

_____

_____

_____

_____

_____

_____

_____

_____

_____

_____

_____

_____

_____

_____

_____

_____

Prompt:

What would your life look like if you believed anything was possible?

Affirmation:

"I am the author of limitless possibility."

_____

_____

_____

_____

_____

_____

_____

_____

_____

_____

_____

_____

_____

_____

_____

_____

_____

_____

_____

_____

Prompt:

What does self-love look and feel like for you?

Affirmation:

"I choose to love myself, every single day."

_____

_____

_____

_____

_____

_____

_____

_____

_____

_____

_____

_____

_____

_____

_____

_____

_____

_____

_____

_____

_____

Visualization & Reprogramming the Mind

You've begun the beautiful work of awareness and reflection. Now, this section invites you to take your healing even deeper.

Your subconscious mind responds to emotion, repetition, and imagery not logic. That means one of the most powerful ways to rewire your inner world is to *see* and *feel* the life you want to create as if it's already yours.

Through the following exercises, you'll visualize your healing, speak your truth, and create new patterns of belief gently and intentionally.

Go slow. Feel into it. Let your imagination become a sanctuary for change.

Guided Visualization: "A Room of Safety"

Close your eyes. Imagine a door in front of you. It can be any shape, size, or color. You feel drawn to open it.

As you step through, you enter a room that is completely yours a place of perfect safety, peace, and love. Every object here supports your healing. The lighting, the smells, the temperature everything is just right.

Take your time to explore. Maybe you find a cozy chair, a soft blanket, or a symbol of strength. Maybe there's music. Or silence. Maybe your future self is sitting here, waiting to greet you.

There may be words written on the walls reminders of truth, beauty, or resilience. Maybe a window opens to a calming landscape or a sky full of stars. A candle glows gently in the corner. The air smells like something comforting lavender, sandalwood, fresh rain.

This room holds no judgment, no pressure, and no fear. It welcomes every part of you: your joy, your grief, your confusion, your clarity. You are safe to cry here. You are safe to laugh here. You are safe to simply be.

Reflection:

What did you see? What did you feel? What will you name this space?

_____

_____

_____

_____

_____

_____

_____

_____

_____

_____

_____

_____

_____

_____

_____

_____

_____

_____

_____

_____

Affirmation Practice

Read each affirmation slowly. Breathe it in. Feel how your body responds. Then, write down the three that speak to you most and say them aloud every day for the next week.

1. I am safe in my body.

2. I am healing, even when it feels invisible.

3. I am worthy of love, without condition.

4. I trust the timing of my journey.

5. I can choose peace in this moment.

6. I am not my thoughts I am the observer.

7. I release what no longer belongs to me.

8. I am enough, exactly as I am.

9. My past does not define my future.

10. I am allowed to rest.

My chosen affirmations:

1._____

2._____

3._____

Rewriting Limiting Beliefs

Write one belief you've been carrying that limits you. Then reframe it into an empowering truth.

Example

Limiting belief: "I'm too broken to be loved."

New belief: "I am lovable, healing, and whole."

Now You Try:

1. Limiting Belief: _____

   New Belief: _____

2. Limiting Belief: _____

   New Belief: _____

3. Limiting Belief: _____

   New Belief: _____

Repeat your new beliefs daily. The more you say them, the more your subconscious mind accepts them.

It might feel strange at first repeating things you don't fully believe yet. That's okay. The old beliefs have been with you for years. They took time to take root, and the new ones will too. But with every repetition, you're laying a new foundation.

Say your affirming beliefs out loud, write them on sticky notes, place them on your mirror or journal page. Let them become familiar. Let them feel like home.

Your subconscious mind learns through repetition and emotion. So the more you pair your new beliefs with feeling hope, peace, self-compassion the deeper they go.

You may not feel a shift overnight. But over time, you'll notice a change: a softer voice inside, a new decision made from worthiness instead of fear, a moment where you chose love over self-doubt.

This is the quiet miracle of reprogramming. Keep going. You are rewiring your truth. You are returning to yourself.

Letter to Your Inner Child

Your inner child still lives within you the younger version of you who needed love, safety, and understanding.

This is your chance to speak to them with the love they always deserved.

Begin your letter here:

Dear little me,

_____

_____

_____

_____

_____

_____

_____

_____

_____

_____

_____

_____

_____

_____

_____

_____

_____

_____

_____

_____

_____

_____

_____

_____

_____

_____

_____

_____

_____

_____

_____

_____

_____

_____

_____

_____

I see you. I love you. You are safe now.

Love,

_____

Designing Your Ideal Day

Let your imagination play. Imagine one full, beautiful day in your life one that reflects healing, joy, peace, and alignment.

Where do you wake up?

What do you see, hear, and feel?

Who are you with (if anyone)?

What do you do?

What makes you smile?

Write it out like a story:

_____

_____

_____

_____

_____

_____

_____

_____

_____

_____

_____

_____

_____

_____

_____

Repetition & Reinforcement Space

Choose one affirmation, new belief, or statement of healing.

Now copy it here **10 times**.

This may seem simple but repetition is how the subconscious mind learns.

_____

_____

_____

_____

_____

_____

_____

_____

_____

_____

_____

_____

_____

_____

_____

_____

_____

_____

You just took a powerful step toward change. Well done.

Season/Milestone Reflections

Healing is not linear. Some months feel like flight. Others feel like fog.

This section is here to help you reflect gently on your progress no matter what it looks like. Whether you come here every season or only after major moments in your life, these reflection pages are your sacred mirror.

They are not about perfection. They are about presence.

Healing doesn't follow a straight path it spirals, deepens, pauses, and sometimes circles back. And that's okay. You are not falling behind. You are unfolding, layer by layer, truth by truth.

Use these pages to notice, not judge. To witness, not rush. To hold space for your wins and your wounds alike.

Come as you are. Return as often as you need.

Even if all you did this month was survive, that matters. Even if you laughed more, cried deeper, loved harder, or simply rested that matters too.

You are always growing, even when it doesn't feel like it. Healing is happening in both the seen and the unseen.

Some growth is loud, like breaking free. Some growth is quiet, like choosing rest. Every step matters. Every moment counts.

Let this be the place where you give yourself credit. Where you pause to honour what you've walked through. Where you offer yourself the grace to be human.

Write it all the messy, the magical, the mundane. Healing happens in the pages we often forget to praise.

This space isn't about doing more. It's about noticing more. Trust that the very act of noticing is a form of healing in itself.

Let these pages witness your truth. Let them remind you of your strength. Let them reflect your becoming.

You are doing beautifully even now.

Spring Reflection Page:

Date: _____

Time: (Season/Milestone) _____

How am I feeling in my body?

_____

_____

_____

_____

_____

_____

_____

_____

_____

_____

_____

_____

_____

_____

_____

_____

_____

_____

_____

_____

What emotions have been present for me lately?

_____

_____

_____

_____

_____

_____

_____

_____

_____

_____

_____

_____

_____

_____

_____

_____

_____

_____

_____

_____

_____

_____

_____

_____

What have I learned about myself?

_____

_____

_____

_____

_____

_____

_____

_____

_____

_____

_____

_____

_____

_____

_____

_____

_____

_____

_____

_____

_____

What did I let go of?

_____

_____

_____

_____

_____

_____

_____

_____

_____

_____

_____

_____

_____

_____

_____

_____

_____

_____

_____

_____

_____

_____

What did I reclaim or remember?

What am I proud of?

What has challenged me?

_____

_____

_____

_____

_____

_____

_____

_____

_____

_____

_____

_____

_____

_____

_____

_____

_____

_____

_____

_____

_____

_____

What do I need more of right now?

Summer Reflection Page:

Date: _____

Time: (Season/Milestone) _____

How am I feeling in my body?

_____

_____

_____

_____

_____

_____

_____

_____

_____

_____

_____

_____

_____

_____

_____

_____

_____

_____

_____

_____

What emotions have been present for me lately?

_____

_____

_____

_____

_____

_____

_____

_____

_____

_____

_____

_____

_____

_____

_____

_____

_____

_____

_____

_____

_____

_____

_____

_____

_____

What have I learned about myself?

_____

_____

_____

_____

_____

_____

_____

_____

_____

_____

_____

_____

_____

_____

_____

_____

_____

_____

_____

_____

_____

_____

What did I let go of?

_____

_____

_____

_____

_____

_____

_____

_____

_____

_____

_____

_____

_____

_____

_____

_____

_____

_____

_____

_____

_____

_____

What did I reclaim or remember?

What am I proud of?

What has challenged me?

_____

_____

_____

_____

_____

_____

_____

_____

_____

_____

_____

_____

_____

_____

_____

_____

_____

_____

_____

_____

What do I need more of right now?

One small step I can take in the next few days:

_____

_____

_____

_____

_____

_____

_____

_____

_____

_____

_____

_____

_____

_____

_____

_____

_____

_____

_____

_____

My intention moving forward:

_____

_____

_____

_____

_____

_____

_____

_____

_____

_____

_____

_____

_____

_____

_____

_____

_____

_____

_____

_____

_____

Fall Reflection Page:

Date: _____

Time: (Season/Milestone) _____

How am I feeling in my body?

_____

_____

_____

_____

_____

_____

_____

_____

_____

_____

_____

_____

_____

_____

_____

_____

_____

_____

_____

_____

_____

_____

What emotions have been present for me lately?

_____

_____

_____

_____

_____

_____

_____

_____

_____

_____

_____

_____

_____

_____

_____

_____

_____

_____

_____

_____

_____

_____

What have I learned about myself?

What did I let go of?

_____

_____

_____

_____

_____

_____

_____

_____

_____

_____

_____

_____

_____

_____

_____

_____

_____

_____

_____

_____

_____

_____

What did I reclaim or remember?

What am I proud of?

_____

_____

_____

_____

_____

_____

_____

_____

_____

_____

_____

_____

_____

_____

_____

_____

_____

_____

_____

_____

_____

_____

_____

_____

What has challenged me?

_____

_____

_____

_____

_____

_____

_____

_____

_____

_____

_____

_____

_____

_____

_____

_____

_____

_____

_____

_____

_____

_____

What do I need more of right now?

_____

_____

_____

_____

_____

_____

_____

_____

_____

_____

_____

_____

_____

_____

_____

_____

_____

_____

_____

_____

_____

_____

One small step I can take in the next few days:

_____

_____

_____

_____

_____

_____

_____

_____

_____

_____

_____

_____

_____

_____

_____

_____

_____

_____

_____

_____

My intention moving forward:

_____

_____

_____

_____

_____

_____

_____

_____

_____

_____

_____

_____

_____

_____

_____

_____

_____

_____

_____

_____

_____

Winter Reflection Page:

Date: _____

Time: (Season/Milestone) _____

How am I feeling in my body?

_____

_____

_____

_____

_____

_____

_____

_____

_____

_____

_____

_____

_____

_____

_____

_____

_____

_____

_____

_____

_____

What emotions have been present for me lately?

_____

_____

_____

_____

_____

_____

_____

_____

_____

_____

_____

_____

_____

_____

_____

_____

_____

_____

_____

_____

_____

What have I learned about myself?

_____

_____

_____

_____

_____

_____

_____

_____

_____

_____

_____

_____

_____

_____

_____

_____

_____

_____

_____

_____

_____

What did I let go of?

_____

_____

_____

_____

_____

_____

_____

_____

_____

_____

_____

_____

_____

_____

_____

_____

_____

_____

_____

_____

_____

_____

_____

What did I reclaim or remember?

_____

_____

_____

_____

_____

_____

_____

_____

_____

_____

_____

_____

_____

_____

_____

_____

_____

_____

_____

_____

_____

What am I proud of?

What has challenged me?

_____

_____

_____

_____

_____

_____

_____

_____

_____

_____

_____

_____

_____

_____

_____

_____

_____

_____

_____

_____

_____

_____

What do I need more of right now?

One small step I can take in the next few days:

_____

_____

_____

_____

_____

_____

_____

_____

_____

_____

_____

_____

_____

_____

_____

_____

_____

_____

_____

_____

_____

My intention moving forward:

_____

_____

_____

_____

_____

_____

_____

_____

_____

_____

_____

_____

_____

_____

_____

_____

_____

_____

_____

_____

_____

Free Creative Space

A Place to Dream, Express, and Just Be

This is your open sky.

There are no rules here only freedom. These pages are yours to fill however, your heart desires.

Draw. Doodle. Scribble. Collage. Vent. Sketch what healing feels like. Create a vision board of your future self. Make a list of things that make you feel alive. Write a poem to your pain. Alternatively, just let your pen wander across the page without needing to explain.

Let your creativity be messy, sacred, beautiful, angry, joyful, confused, whatever it is, let it be real.

You don't need to be an artist to express yourself. You don't need to be perfect to belong here. What matters is showing up for yourself with honesty and care.

How You Might Use This Space

Consider using this space to:

- Track your emotional patterns with color

- Create mandalas for focus and calm

- Write letters you'll never send

- Sketch your "before and after" healing

- Draw symbols or images that bring you peace

- Start a gratitude collage with meaningful words or images

DRAWING & CREATIVE PAGES

Draw what healing looks like today.

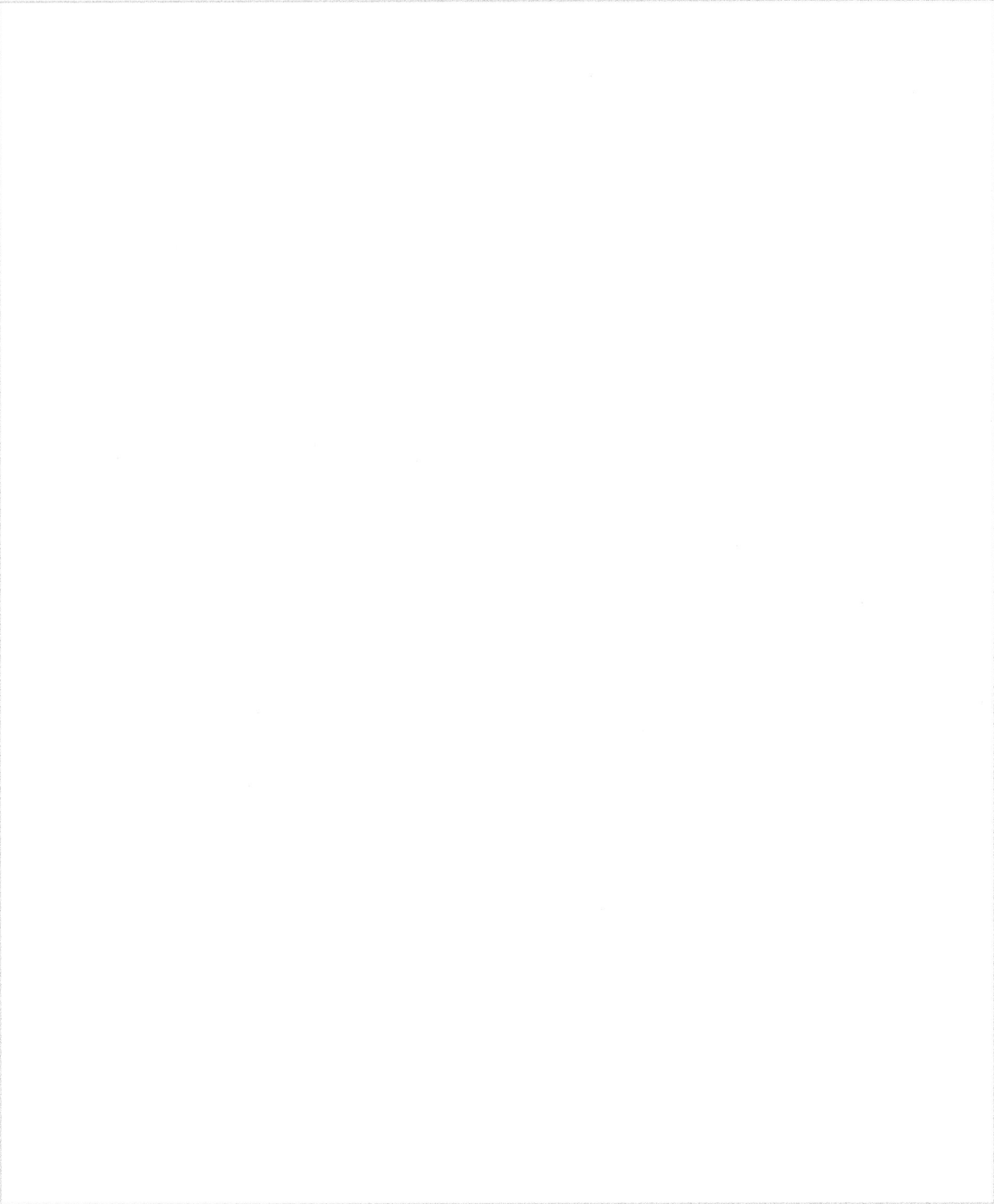

Sketch your safe space, dream home, or sanctuary.

Use symbols, shapes, or colors to express your emotions

VISION BOARD PAGES

"Paste images that represent your goals"

"Include colors, textures, and quotes that inspire you"

"Let your imagination lead the way"

"My Vision Board"

"My Vision Board"

"My Vision Board"

WRITING PAGES

Speak Freely

_____

_____

_____

_____

_____

_____

_____

_____

_____

_____

_____

_____

_____

_____

_____

_____

_____

_____

_____

_____

_____

_____

_____

_____

_____

_____

_____

Whatever Needs to Come Through

Untangle What You're Feeling

Write to Release

A Letter to Myself Today

_____

_____

_____

_____

_____

_____

_____

_____

_____

_____

_____

_____

_____

_____

_____

_____

_____

_____

_____

_____

_____

_____

Final Reflection Prompt:

"Who Have I Become?

This is your mirror.

You've walked through awareness, release, rewriting, and creative self-expression. Now, take a moment to witness yourself without judgment. Who are you now? What has softened in you? What has grown stronger?

This is your invitation to acknowledge your own becoming.

You've turned inward, you've listened, and you've shown up for your pain, your dreams, your truth. That matters. Whether your steps were bold or quiet, whether your progress was visible or internal, it was all part of your healing.

Now, Pause. Breathe.

You may not be exactly where you want to be but you are no longer, where you once were. Growth isn't always loud. Sometimes it's the simple fact that you kept going.

Look at yourself with kind eyes.

What have you discovered about your heart, your voice, your resilience?

This is your mirror moment. Let it reflect your strength, your softness, and your beautiful, unfolding self.

You are becoming. In addition, you are already enough.

Now, look forward. What parts of you are ready to lead the way? What new truths will you walk with from here?

This page is yours to celebrate who you've become and who you're still becoming.

Write freely. Let it be a love letter to yourself.

Affirmations to Carry Forward

Anchor your truth.

Let these affirmations become your daily touchstones. Say them. Write them. Breathe them in. You may even add your own.

These words are more than thoughts they are reminders, invitations, and seeds of truth that your heart already knows. The more you repeat them, the more your subconscious mind will believe them. Over time, they begin to rewire your inner narrative, soften self-doubt, and anchor you in compassion.

Speak them in the mirror. Whisper them when you wake. Write them on sticky notes, journal pages, or the corners of your to-do lists. Let them live in your space, in your breath, in your being.

In addition, when old stories rise up again because they will return to these affirmations like you would to a safe harbor. They are here for you. They are yours now.

Choose the ones that feel true. Choose the ones that feel hard. Then repeat them anyway.

You are worthy of every word.

Examples:

☐ I am safe to take up space.

☐ I trust the rhythm of my healing.

☐ I deserve to feel peace in my body.

☐ I release guilt and invite grace.

☐ I am allowed to change.

☐ I am whole, even when I'm still healing.

☐ My voice matters.

☐ I am enough.

☐ I forgive myself daily.

☐ I am becoming more of who I truly am.

Place approx. 10 total on the page

_____

_____

_____

_____

_____

_____

_____

_____

_____

_____

_____

_____

Letter to Your Future Self

Letter to My Future Self

Speak to the one who's still becoming.

Imagine yourself six months or one year from now. What would you want them to remember? What do you hope they've continued? Write from the heart, without needing to sound wise or perfect. This is your message to the version of you still growing forward.

Take this opportunity to speak with love, honesty, and hope. What have you learned that you don't want to forget? What encouragement can you offer from where you are right now? What dreams do you hope they've pursued, and what habits do you hope they've let go of?

Let this letter become a bridge between your present self and your future self a message that says, "You matter. I believe in you. Keep going."

You may want to include the things you're proud of, the healing you've done, and the parts of yourself you hope they've grown into. You might even remind them of your struggles not to dwell, but to honor how far you've come.

This is more than just a letter it's a conversation across time. It's a chance to remind yourself of your strength, your values, your goals, and your growth. What do you hope they've forgiven? What boundaries do you want them to honor? What kind of love do you hope they've allowed into their life?

You can include words of reassurance, or even a list of promises to yourself. Let it be honest, even if it's vulnerable. There's no right way to write this letter only your way.

Let it carry your voice forward like a light in the dark.

Speak gently. Dream boldly.

Your future self is already listening.

Optional Note:

You can date this letter, seal it, or return to it on a specific day. Let this be a time capsule of your healing.

108

Dear Future Me Letter Page

Dear Future Me,

_____

_____

_____

_____

_____

_____

_____

_____

_____

_____

_____

_____

_____

_____

With love,

_____

Sign your name here: _____

Revisit this letter on _____